Table of Contents

INTRODUCTION

Weight loss experts still recommend low-carb diets as the most effective way to shed pounds. While reducing both calories and carbs might seem like a winning strategy for weight loss, excessively cutting carbs can actually hinder progress. There's ongoing debate about the necessary carb intake for weight loss, suggesting that extreme reductions as seen in keto and Whole30 diets aren't essential. This 30-day low-carb meal plan provides tasty recipes for breakfast, lunch, and dinner, illustrating a healthy approach to weight reduction without extreme carb restrictions.

Since many fiber-rich foods like whole grains, legumes, certain fruits, and starchy vegetables are high in carbohydrates, reducing these foods can inadvertently lower fiber intake. Maintaining adequate fiber consumption is crucial for feeling full and satisfied after meals.

Carbohydrates also provide essential nutrients such as vitamin D and calcium, particularly abundant in dairy products. Therefore, this meal plan minimizes carbs while ensuring these vital nutrients aren't neglected. Healthy carb sources like fruit, Greek yogurt, and beans remain part of the plan.

Research indicates that adopting a low-calorie, low-carb diet can aid weight loss. However, it's unnecessary to follow extreme carb restrictions like those in Atkins or ketogenic diets to achieve weight loss. In fact, insufficient carb intake may impede weight loss by depriving the body of essential nutrients and fiber, which contribute to satiety on fewer calories.

This straightforward low-carb meal plan maintains a balanced intake of essential elements without sacrificing nutrition. Additionally, it prioritizes sufficient daily protein intake (nearly 50 grams) to promote fullness while consuming fewer calories and carbs. Following this low-carb, high-protein meal plan can help you lose a healthy 1 to 2 pounds per week at 1,200 calories per day.

1200 CALORIE LOW CARB MEAL PLAN

Day 1

Breakfast (201 calories, 14 g carbohydrates)

- 1 cup nonfat plain Greek yogurt

- 1/3 cup blackberries

- 1 Tbsp. chopped walnuts

A.M. Snack (70 calories, 18 g carbohydrates)

- 2 clementines

Lunch (360 calories, 30 g carbohydrates)

- 1 serving White Bean & Veggie Salad

P.M. Snack (32 calories, 7 g carbohydrates)

- 1/2 cup raspberries

Dinner (555 calories, 37 g carbohydrates)

- 1 serving Ginger-Tahini Oven-Baked Salmon & Vegetables

Daily Totals: 1,218 calories, 75 g protein, 106 g carbohydrates, 30 g fiber, 61 g fat, 1,123 mg sodium

Day 2

Breakfast (288 calories, 22 g carbohydrates)

- 1 serving Greek Muffin-Tin Omelets with Feta & Peppers

- 1 medium orange

A.M. Snack (131 calories, 35 g carbohydrates)

- 1 large pear

Lunch (344 calories, 47 g carbohydrates)

- 1 serving Chipotle-Lime Cauliflower Taco Bowls

P.M. Snack (51 calories, 10 g carbohydrates)

- 1 large bell pepper, sliced

Dinner (394 calories, 14 g carbohydrates)

- 1 serving Homemade Chicken Tenders with Everything Bagel Seasoning over Salad

Breakfast (288 calories, 22 g carbohydrates)

• 1 serving Greek Muffin-Tin Omelets with Feta & Peppers

• 1 medium orange

A.M. Snack (35 calories, 9 g carbohydrates)

• 1 clementine

Lunch (344 calories, 47 g carbohydrates)

• 1 serving Chipotle-Lime Cauliflower Taco Bowls

P.M. Snack (131 calories, 35 g carbohydrates)

• 1 large pear

Dinner (411 calories, 25 g carbohydrates)

• 1 serving Chicken Cutlets with Sun-Dried Tomato Cream Sauce

• 2 cups steamed broccoli florets

Meal-Prep Tip: Prepare 2 servings Blueberry Almond Chia Pudding to have for breakfast on Days 4 & 5.

Daily Totals: 1,209 calories, 63 g protein, 138 g carbohydrates, 36 g fiber, 50 g fat, 1344 mg sodium

Day 4

Breakfast (229 calories, 30 g carbohydrates)

• 1 serving Blueberry Almond Chia Pudding

A.M. Snack (35 calories, 9 g carbohydrates)

• 1 clementine

Lunch (344 calories, 47 g carbohydrates)

• 1 serving Chipotle-Lime Cauliflower Taco Bowls

P.M. Snack (226 calories, 7 g carbohydrates)

• 1 serving Greek Muffin-Tin Omelets with Feta & Peppers

Dinner (376 calories, 21 g carbohydrates)

• 1 serving Sheet-Pan Maple-Mustard Pork Chops & Carrots

Daily Totals: 1,210 calories, 57 g protein, 114 g carbohydrates, 30 g fiber, 62 g fat, 1,552 mg sodium

Breakfast (229 calories, 30 g carbohydrates)

• 1 serving Blueberry Almond Chia Pudding

A.M. Snack (66 calories, 4 g carbohydrates)

• 1/2 cup nonfat plain Greek yogurt

Lunch (344 calories, 47 g carbohydrates)

• 1 serving Chipotle-Lime Cauliflower Taco Bowls

P.M. Snack (77 calories, 3 g carbohydrates)

• 10 dry-roasted unsalted almonds

Dinner (490 calories, 27 g carbohydrates)

• 1 serving No-Noodle Eggplant Lasagna

• 1 serving Traditional Greek Salad

Meal-Prep Tip: Reserve 2 servings of the No-Noodle Eggplant Lasagna to have for lunch on Days 6 & 7.

Daily Totals: 1,206 calories, 61 g protein, 111 g carbohydrates, 32 g fiber, 61 g fat, 1,502 mg sodium

Breakfast (201 calories, 14 g carbohydrates)

- 1 cup nonfat plain Greek yogurt

- 1/3 cup blackberries

- 1 Tbsp. chopped walnuts

A.M. Snack (131 calories, 35 g carbohydrates)

- 1 large pear

Lunch (348 calories, 30 g carbohydrates)

- 1 serving No-Noodle Eggplant Lasagna

- 1/3 cup pomegranate seeds

P.M. Snack (116 calories, 31 g carbohydrates)

- 1 large apple

Dinner (428 calories, 17 g carbohydrates)

- 1 serving Thai Tofu & Vegetable Curry with Zucchini Noodles

Daily Totals: 1,224 calories, 67 g protein, 127 g carbohydrates, 29 g fiber, 57 g fat, 1,012 mg sodium

Breakfast (288 calories, 22 g carbohydrates)

- 1 serving Greek Muffin-Tin Omelets with Feta & Peppers

- 1 medium orange

A.M. Snack (50 calories, 12 g carbohydrates)

- 2 medium carrots, sliced

Lunch (337 calories, 26 g carbohydrates)

- 1 serving No-Noodle Eggplant Lasagna

- 1 medium bell pepper, sliced

P.M. Snack (131 calories, 35 g carbohydrates)

- 1 large pear

Dinner (413 calories, 13 g carbohydrates)

- 1 serving Shrimp Cauliflower Fried Rice

- 2 cups mixed greens

- 1 serving Homemade Vinaigrette with Sesame & Ginger

Breakfast: 1 serving (2 mini omelets) Easy Loaded Baked Omelet Muffins and 1 medium orange (273 calories, 20 g carbs)

• A.M. Snack: 1 cup blackberries (62 calories, 14 g carbs)

Lunch: 1 serving White Bean & Veggie Salad (360 calories, 30 g carbs)

• P.M. Snack: 1 medium apple (95 calories, 25 g carbs)

Dinner: 1 serving Korean Steak, Kimchi & Cauliflower Rice Bowls (414 calories, 20 g carbs)

Daily Totals: 1,204 calories, 60 g protein, 109 g carbohydrates, 35 g fiber, 63 g fat, 1,531 mg sodium.

Day 9

• Breakfast: 1 serving (2 mini omelets) Easy Loaded Baked Omelet Muffins and 1 medium orange (273 calories, 20 g carbs)

• A.M. Snack: 1 cup raspberries topped with 1/4 cup whole-milk plain Greek yogurt & 1 tsp. chia seeds (143 calories, 19 g carbs)

• Lunch: 1 serving Zucchini Noodles with Quick Turkey Bolognese (216 calories, 16 g carbs)

• P.M. Snack: 1 medium apple and 6 almonds (141 calories, 27 calories)

• Dinner: 1 serving One-Pot Garlicky Shrimp & Spinach with 1 (3-inch) slice whole-wheat baguette, toasted and drizzled with 1 tsp. olive oil (448 calories, 45 g carbs)

Daily Totals: 1,220 calories, 78 g protein, 126 g carbohydrates, 27 g fiber, 51 g fat, 1,916 mg sodium.

Day 10

• Breakfast: 1 serving Two-Ingredient Banana Pancakes topped with 1 Tbsp. maple syrup & 1 cup blackberries (238 calories, 41 g carbs)

• A.M. Snack: 2 plums and 12 almonds (153 calories, 18 g carbs)

• Lunch: 1 serving Zucchini Noodles with Quick Turkey Bolognese and 1 medium orange (278 calories, 31 g carbs)

• P.M. Snack: 3 cups air-popped popcorn drizzled with 1 tsp. olive oil & a pinch of salt (135 calories, 18 g carbs)

• Dinner: 1 serving Guacamole Chicken with 1 serving Mexican Cauliflower Rice (397 calories, 13 g carbs)

Daily Totals: 1,201 calories, 64 g protein, 122 g carbohydrates, 29 g fiber, 57 g fat, 1,531 mg sodium.

Day 11

• Breakfast: 1 serving (2 mini omelets) Easy Loaded Baked Omelet Muffins and 1 medium orange (273 calories, 20 g carbs)

• A.M. Snack: 1 cup blackberries and 10 almonds (139 calories, 17 g carbs)

• Lunch: 1 serving Zucchini Noodles with Quick Turkey Bolognese and 1 medium apple (311 calories, 41 g carbs)

• P.M. Snack: 1 medium pear (101 calories, 27 g carbs)

• Dinner: 1 serving each Walnut-Rosemary Crusted Salmon and Roasted Broccoli with Lemon Garlic Vinaigrette (389 calories, 12 g carbs)

Daily Totals: 1,213 calories, 69 g protein, 117 g carbohydrates, 29 g fiber, 59 g fat, 1,558 mg sodium.

Day 12

• Breakfast: 1 serving Two-Ingredient Banana Pancakes topped with 1 Tbsp. maple syrup & 1 cup blackberries (238 calories, 41 g carbs)

• A.M. Snack: 1 medium pear and 10 almonds (179 calories, 30 g carbs)

• Lunch: 1 serving Zucchini Noodles with Quick Turkey Bolognese (216 calories, 16 g carbs)

• P.M. Snack: 1 medium apple and 1 1/2 oz. Cheddar cheese (266 calories, 26 g carbs)

• Dinner: 1 serving Cauliflower Mac & Cheese with 1/4 cup peas & 1 sliced cooked bacon mixed in (316 calories, 16 g carbs)

• Meal-Prep Tip: Refrigerate 1 serving of the mac & cheese with peas & bacon to have for lunch on Day 13.

Daily Totals: 1,215 calories, 59 g protein, 129 g carbohydrates, 27 g fiber, 58 g fat, 1,568 mg sodium.

Day 13

• Breakfast: 1 cup raspberries topped with 1/2 cup whole-milk plain Greek yogurt, 1 tsp. chia seeds & 1 Tbsp. each shredded unsweetened coconut & slivered almonds (277 calories, 24 g carbs)

• A.M. Snack: 1 medium orange (62 calories, 15 g carbs)

• Lunch: 1 serving Cauliflower Mac & Cheese with 1/4 cup peas and 1 sliced cooked bacon mixed in (316 calories, 16 g carbs)

• P.M. Snack: 1 medium apple and 1 oz. Cheddar cheese (209 calories, 26 g carbs)

• Dinner: 1 serving Broiled Ginger-Lime Chicken with 1 serving Tequila Guacamole (336 calories, 10 g carbs)

- Meal-Prep Tip: Refrigerate 1 serving of the chicken and guacamole to have for lunch on Day 14.

Daily Totals: 1,200 calories, 64 g protein, 92 g carbohydrates, 28 g fiber, 69 g fat, 1,469 mg sodium.

Day 14

- Breakfast: "Egg in a Hole" Peppers with Avocado Salsa (285 calories, 14 g carbs)

- A.M. Snack: 1 cup raspberries topped with 1/3 cup whole-milk plain Greek yogurt & 1 tsp. chia seeds (162 calories, 20 g carbs)

- Lunch: 1 serving Broiled Ginger-Lime Chicken with 1 serving Tequila Guacamole (336 calories, 10 g carbs)

- P.M. Snack: 1 medium orange (62 calories, 15 g carbs)

- Dinner: 1 serving Slow-Cooker Vegetable Soup with 1 (3-inch) slice whole-wheat baguette (355 calories, 65 g carbs)

- Meal-Prep Tip: Refrigerate 2 servings of the soup to have for lunch on Day 15. Freeze 3 single servings of the soup in individual containers to have for lunch on Days 20, 21 and 29.

Daily Totals: 1,200 calories, 66 g protein, 125 g carbohydrates, 33 g fiber, 54 g fat, 2,318 mg sodium.

1200 CALORIE LOW CARB COOKBOOK

Shrimp and Veggie Stuffed Zucchini

Ingredients

1 extra large zucchini

4 tablespoons olive oil, divided

6 cloves garlic, finely chopped

1 shallot, finely chopped

½ pound large shrimp - shelled, deveined, and cut in half

1 large tomato - peeled, seeded and diced

8 cremini mushrooms, quartered

¼ cup grated Parmesan cheese

8 leaves fresh basil, torn

ground black pepper to taste

kosher salt to taste

garlic powder to taste

4 tablespoons grated Parmesan cheese, divided

Directions

Preheat the oven's broiler and set the oven rack about 6 inches from the heat source. Grease a baking sheet.

Cut zucchini in half lengthwise and scoop out seeds and pulp, leaving a thick shell of flesh. Brush both halves of zucchini with 1 tablespoon olive oil and place them cut-side down onto the prepared baking sheet. Bake until zucchini is hot and beginning to release beads of moisture, 5 to 10 minutes. Remove zucchini from the oven.

Preheat the oven to 450 degrees F (230 degrees C).

Heat 2 tablespoons olive oil in a skillet over medium-low heat. Cook and stir garlic and shallot until translucent, about 5 minutes. Remove from heat and let cool.

Place remaining 1 tablespoon olive oil, shrimp, tomato, mushrooms, 1/4 cup Parmesan cheese, basil, and cooked garlic and shallot into a bowl, and stir to mix. Season with salt, pepper, and garlic powder. Stuff the mixture into zucchini halves, and sprinkle each zucchini with about 2 tablespoons Parmesan cheese.

Bake stuffed zucchini in the preheated oven until cheese is browned and filling is cooked through and hot, about 20 minutes.

White Bean & Veggie Salad

Ingredients

• 2 cups mixed salad greens

• ¾ cup veggies of your choice, such as chopped cucumbers and cherry tomatoes

21

- ⅓ cup canned white beans, rinsed and drained

- ½ avocado, diced

- 1 tablespoon red-wine vinegar

- 2 teaspoons extra-virgin olive oil

- ¼ teaspoon kosher salt

- Freshly ground pepper to taste

Directions

- Combine greens, veggies, beans and avocado in a medium bowl. Drizzle with vinegar and oil and season with salt and pepper. Toss to combine and transfer to a large plate.

Ginger-Tahini Oven-Baked Salmon & Vegetables

Ingredients

- 1 large sweet potato, cubed (about 12 oz.)

- 1 pound white button or cremini mushrooms, cut into 1-inch pieces (6 cups)

- 2 tablespoons olive oil, divided

- ½ teaspoon salt, divided

- 1 pound green beans, trimmed

- 2 tablespoons reduced-sodium soy sauce

- 1 tablespoon plus 2 tsp. tahini

- 1 tablespoon plus 1 tsp. honey

- 1 ½ teaspoons finely grated fresh ginger

- 1 ¼ pounds salmon, preferably wild-caught, cut into 4 portions

- 2 teaspoons rice vinegar

- 2 tablespoons chopped fresh chives (Optional)

Directions

- Place a large rimmed baking sheet in the oven. Position one rack in the middle of the oven and another about 6 inches from the broiler. Preheat to 425 degrees F.

23

- Combine sweet potato, mushrooms, 1 Tbsp. oil, and 1/4 tsp. salt in a large bowl; toss to coat.

- Remove the baking sheet from the oven. Spread the vegetable mixture in an even layer on the pan; roast, stirring once, until the sweet potatoes are starting to brown, about 20 minutes.

- Meanwhile, toss green beans with the remaining 1 Tbsp. oil and 1/4 tsp. salt. Combine soy sauce, tahini, honey, and ginger in a small bowl.

- Remove the pan from the oven. Move the mushrooms and sweet potatoes to one side and place the green beans on the other side. Place salmon in the middle, nestling it on top of the vegetables, if necessary. Spread half of the tahini sauce on top of the salmon. Roast until the salmon flakes, 8 to 10 minutes more. Turn broiler to high; move the pan to the top rack and broil until the salmon is glazed, about 3 minutes.

- Stir vinegar into the remaining tahini sauce and drizzle it over the salmon and vegetables. Garnish with chives, if desired, and serve.

Ingredients

- Cooking spray

- 2 tablespoons extra-virgin olive oil

- ¾ cup diced onion

- ¼ teaspoon salt, divided

- 1 medium red bell pepper, diced

- 1 tablespoon finely chopped fresh oregano

- 8 large eggs

- ¾ cup crumbled feta cheese

- ½ cup low-fat milk

- ½ teaspoon ground pepper

- 2 cups chopped fresh spinach

- ¼ cup sliced Kalamata olives

Directions

• Preheat oven to 325 degrees F. Liberally coat a 12-cup muffin tin with cooking spray.

• Heat oil in a large skillet over medium heat. Add onion and 1/8 teaspoon salt; cook, stirring, until starting to soften, about 3 minutes. Add bell pepper and oregano; cook, stirring, until the vegetables are tender and starting to brown, 4 to 5 minutes more. Remove from heat and let cool for 5 minutes.

• Whisk eggs, feta, milk, pepper and the remaining 1/8 teaspoon salt in a large bowl. Stir in spinach, olives and the vegetable mixture. Divide among the prepared muffin cups.

• Bake until firm to the touch, about 25 minutes. Let stand for 5 minutes before removing from the tin.

Chipotle-Lime Cauliflower Taco Bowls

Ingredients

• ¼ cup lime juice (from about 2 limes)

• 1-2 tablespoons chopped chipotles in adobo sauce

• 1 tablespoon honey

- 2 cloves garlic

- ½ teaspoon salt

- 1 small head cauliflower, cut into bite-size pieces

- 1 small red onion, halved and thinly sliced

- 2 cups cooked quinoa, cooled

- 1 cup no-salt-added canned black beans, rinsed

- ½ cup crumbled queso fresco

- 1 cup shredded red cabbage

- 1 medium avocado

- 1 lime, cut into 4 wedges (Optional)

Directions

- Preheat oven to 450°F. Line a large rimmed baking sheet with foil.

- Combine lime juice, chipotles to taste, honey, garlic and salt in a blender. Process until mostly smooth. Place cauliflower in a large bowl; add the sauce and stir to coat.

Transfer to the prepared baking sheet. Sprinkle onion over the cauliflower. Roast, stirring once, until the cauliflower is tender and browned in spots, 18 to 20 minutes; set aside to cool.

• Divide quinoa among 4 single-serving lidded containers (1/2 cup each). Top each with one-fourth of the cauliflower mixture, 1/4 cup black beans and 2 tablespoons cheese. Seal the containers and refrigerate for up to 4 days.

• To reheat 1 container, vent the lid and microwave on High until steaming, 2 1/2 to 3 minutes. Top with 1/4 cup cabbage and 1/4 avocado (sliced). Serve with a lime wedge, if desired.

Homemade Chicken Tenders with Everything Bagel Seasoning over Salad

Ingredients

• 2 tablespoons all-purpose flour

• 1 large egg

• ½ cup panko breadcrumbs, preferably whole-wheat

• 1 tablespoon everything bagel seasoning

- 1 pound chicken tenders

- ¼ cup grapeseed or canola oil

- 2 tablespoons extra-virgin olive oil

- 1 tablespoon white-wine vinegar

- 1 teaspoon Dijon mustard

- 1 teaspoon honey

- ⅛ teaspoon ground pepper

- 5 ounces mixed baby greens

Directions

- Place flour in a shallow dish and lightly beat egg in another shallow dish. Mix breadcrumbs and everything bagel seasoning in a third shallow dish. Dredge chicken tenders in flour, then egg, then breadcrumbs.

- Heat grapeseed (or canola) oil in a large skillet over medium-high heat. Add the chicken and cook, turning once, until golden brown and an instant-read thermometer

29

registers 165 degrees F, about 7 minutes total, adjusting the heat as needed to prevent burning.

• Whisk olive oil, vinegar, mustard, honey and pepper in a large bowl. Add greens and toss to coat. Serve the greens topped with the chicken.

Chicken Cutlets with Sun-Dried Tomato Cream Sauce

Ingredients

• 1 pound chicken cutlets

• ¼ teaspoon salt, divided

• ¼ teaspoon ground pepper, divided

• ½ cup slivered oil-packed sun-dried tomatoes, plus 1 tablespoon oil from the jar

• ½ cup finely chopped shallots

• ½ cup dry white wine

• ½ cup heavy cream

• 2 tablespoons chopped fresh parsley

Directions

• Sprinkle chicken with 1/8 teaspoon each salt and pepper. Heat sun-dried tomato oil in a large skillet over medium heat. Add the chicken and cook, turning once, until browned and an instant-read thermometer inserted into the thickest part registers 165°F, about 6 minutes total. Transfer to a plate.

• Add sun-dried tomatoes and shallots to the pan. Cook, stirring, for 1 minute. Increase heat to high and add wine. Cook, scraping up any browned bits, until the liquid has mostly evaporated, about 2 minutes. Reduce heat to medium and stir in cream, any accumulated juices from the chicken and the remaining 1/8 teaspoon each salt and pepper; simmer for 2 minutes. Return the chicken to the pan and turn to coat with the sauce. Serve the chicken topped with the sauce and parsley.

Blueberry Almond Chia Pudding

Ingredients

• ½ cup unsweetened almond milk or other nondairy milk beverage

• 2 tablespoons chia seeds

• 2 teaspoons pure maple syrup

• ⅛ teaspoon almond extract

• ½ cup fresh blueberries, divided

• 1 tablespoon toasted slivered almonds, divided

Directions

• Stir together almond milk (or other nondairy milk beverage), chia, maple syrup and almond extract in a small bowl. Cover and refrigerate for at least 8 hours and up to 3 days.

• When ready to serve, stir the pudding well. Spoon about half the pudding into a serving glass (or bowl) and top with half the blueberries and almonds. Add the rest of the pudding and top with the remaining blueberries and almonds.

Sheet-Pan Maple-Mustard Pork Chops & Carrots

Ingredients

- 4 tablespoons extra-virgin olive oil, divided

- 1 tablespoon whole-grain mustard

- 1 tablespoon maple syrup

- 4 (5 ounce) bone-in, center-cut pork chops (1/2 inch thick)

- 1 ½ pounds rainbow carrots, cut diagonally into 1/4-inch slices

- 2 teaspoons finely chopped garlic

- 1 teaspoon coarsely chopped peeled fresh ginger

- ½ teaspoon ground turmeric

- ¾ teaspoon kosher salt

- ¾ teaspoon ground pepper

- ¼ cup chopped flat-leaf parsley

Directions

• Position a rack in the lower third of the oven and preheat to 450 degrees F.

• Whisk 1 tablespoon oil, mustard and maple syrup in a small bowl. Place pork chops on one side of a rimmed baking sheet. Brush the tops with the oil mixture. Place carrots on the other side and drizzle with the remaining 3 tablespoons oil. Sprinkle garlic, ginger and turmeric on the carrots and toss to coat. Season everything with salt and pepper. Roast for 10 minutes.

• Turn broiler to high. Broil until an instant-read thermometer inserted in the thickest part of a chop without touching the bone registers 145 degrees F, about 4 minutes. Continue cooking the carrots, if needed, until tender and glazed, 2 to 5 minutes more. Serve sprinkled with parsley.

No-Noodle Eggplant Lasagna

Ingredients

• 2 large eggplants (2 1/2-3 pounds total), cut lengthwise into 1/4-inch thick slices

- 1 tablespoon extra-virgin olive oil

- 12 ounces lean ground beef

- 1 cup chopped onion

- 2 cloves garlic, minced

- 1 (28 ounce) can no-salt-added crushed tomatoes

- ¼ cup dry red wine

- 1 teaspoon dried basil

- 1 teaspoon dried oregano

- ¾ teaspoon salt

- ¼ teaspoon ground pepper

- 1 ½ cups part-skim ricotta cheese

- 1 large egg, lightly beaten

- 1 cup shredded part-skim mozzarella cheese, divided

- Chopped fresh basil for garnish

Directions

- Preheat oven to 400 degrees F. Coat 2 large baking sheets with cooking spray.

- Arrange eggplant slices in a single layer on the prepared pans. Roast until just tender, 15 to 20 minutes.

- Meanwhile, heat oil in a large skillet over medium-high heat. Add beef and onion; cook, stirring and crumbling with a wooden spoon, until browned, 6 to 8 minutes. Add garlic; cook for 1 minute. Add tomatoes, wine, basil, oregano, salt and pepper; bring to a simmer. Reduce heat to medium-low and cook, stirring occasionally, until thickened, about 10 minutes.

- Combine ricotta and egg in a small bowl.

- Spread about 1 cup of the sauce in a 9-by-13-inch baking dish. Arrange 1/4 of the eggplant slices over the tomato sauce. Dollop on about 1/3 cup of the ricotta mixture and sprinkle with 1/4 cup mozzarella. Make another layer with another 1/4 of the eggplant slices, this time arranging them crosswise to the first layer. Top with 1 cup sauce, dollop on 1/3 cup ricotta mixture and sprinkle with 1/4 cup mozzarella. Repeat with the remaining ingredients to make 2 more layers.

36

• Bake the lasagna, uncovered, until the sauce is bubbling around the edges, 30 to 40 minutes. Let stand for 10 to 20 minutes before serving. Garnish with fresh basil, if desired.

Traditional Greek Salad

Ingredients

• 3 tablespoons extra-virgin olive oil

• 1 tablespoon lemon juice

• 1 tablespoon red-wine vinegar

• 1 teaspoon dried oregano

• ¼ teaspoon salt

• ¼ teaspoon ground pepper

• 2 ripe medium tomatoes, cut into 3/4-inch dice

• 1 ½ cups diced cucumber (3/4-inch)

• 1 cup diced green bell pepper (3/4-inch)

• ⅓ cup thinly sliced red onion

• ¼ cup quartered pitted Kalamata olives

• ½ cup diced feta cheese (2 1/2 ounces)

Directions

• Whisk oil, lemon juice, vinegar, oregano, salt and pepper together in a large bowl. Add tomatoes, cucumber, bell pepper, onion, olives and feta. Toss to coat.

Tofu & Vegetable Curry with Zucchini Noodles

Ingredients

• 2 tablespoons toasted sesame oil

• 1 (14 ounce) package extra-firm tofu, cut into 1/2-inch pieces

• 1 (14 ounce) can coconut milk

• 2 tablespoons red curry paste

• 1 tablespoon lime juice

- 2 medium cloves garlic, grated

- ½ teaspoon salt

- 1 tablespoon avocado oil

- 1 (8 ounce) package sliced mushrooms

- 1 bunch scallions, cut into 1-inch pieces

- 6 cups chopped kale

- 2 (10 ounce) packages zucchini noodles

Directions

- Heat sesame oil in a large nonstick skillet over medium-high heat. Pat tofu dry and add to pan. Cook in a single layer, without stirring, until the pieces turn golden, about 4 minutes. Gently stir and continue cooking, stirring occasionally, until golden all over, 4 minutes more. Transfer to a plate.

- Meanwhile, whisk coconut milk, curry paste, lime juice, garlic and salt in a small bowl.

• Add avocado oil, mushrooms and scallions to the pan. Cook, stirring, until the mushrooms have released their liquid and started to brown, about 5 minutes. Add kale, the sauce mixture and the tofu and cook, stirring, until the kale is wilted, the sauce has thickened and the tofu is heated through, about 2 minutes. Transfer to a bowl.

• Add zucchini noodles to the pan and cook, stirring, until heated through, about 1 minute. Serve the curry over the noodles.

Shrimp Cauliflower Fried Rice

Ingredients

• ¼ cup sesame oil, divided

• 2 large eggs, lightly beaten

• 3 cups riced cauliflower

• 1 pound large shrimp (31-35 count), peeled and deveined

• 3 cups broccoli florets

• 1 medium red bell pepper, thinly sliced (about 1 cup)

- 3 cloves garlic, sliced

- 3 tablespoons reduced-sodium soy sauce or tamari

- 2 tablespoons water

- 1 tablespoon rice vinegar

- ½ teaspoon ground pepper

Directions

- Heat 2 teaspoons oil in a large flat-bottomed carbon-steel wok or large, heavy skillet over high heat. Add eggs and cook, without stirring, until fully cooked on one side, about 30 seconds. Flip and cook until just cooked through, about 15 seconds. Transfer to a cutting board and cut into 1/2-inch pieces.

- Add 2 teaspoons oil to the pan; heat over high heat. Add cauliflower in an even layer; cook, undisturbed, until lightly browned, 3 to 4 minutes. Transfer to a plate.

- Add 2 teaspoons oil to the pan; heat over high heat. Add shrimp; cook, stirring often, until just opaque, about 3 minutes. Transfer to the plate with the cauliflower.

41

• Add the remaining 2 tablespoons oil to the pan; heat over high heat. Add broccoli, bell pepper and garlic; cook, stirring occasionally, until lightly charred, 4 to 5 minutes. Stir in soy sauce (or tamari), water, vinegar and pepper. Bring to a boil; boil for 30 seconds. Remove from the heat. Stir in the reserved eggs, cauliflower and shrimp.

Homemade Vinaigrette with Sesame & Ginger

Ingredients

• ½ cup grapeseed oil

• ¼ cup rice vinegar

• 2 teaspoons minced scallions

• 1 teaspoon minced fresh ginger

• 1 teaspoon sesame oil

• 1 teaspoon honey

• ¾ teaspoon salt

Directions

42

• Pour grapeseed oil into a mason jar. Add vinegar, scallions, ginger, sesame oil, honey and salt. Cover and shake to blend.

Low-Carb Bacon & Broccoli Egg Burrito

Ingredients

• 1 slice bacon

• 1 cup chopped broccoli

• ¼ cup chopped tomato

• 1 large egg

• 1 tablespoon reduced-fat milk

• 1 scallion, sliced

• ⅛ teaspoon salt

• ⅛ teaspoon ground pepper

• 1 teaspoon canola or avocado oil

• 2 tablespoons shredded sharp Cheddar cheese

Directions

• Cook bacon in a medium nonstick skillet over medium heat, turning once or twice, until crisp, 4 to 6 minutes. Remove to a paper towel-lined plate. Add broccoli to the pan and cook, stirring, until soft, about 3 minutes. Stir in tomato and transfer to a small bowl.

• Meanwhile, whisk egg, milk, scallion, salt and pepper in another bowl. When the vegetables are cooked, wipe out the skillet. Add oil and heat over medium heat. Add the egg mixture, tilting to coat the bottom of the pan. Cook, undisturbed, until set on the bottom, about 2 minutes. Using a thin, wide silicone spatula, carefully flip the egg "tortilla." Sprinkle with cheese and cook until completely set, about 1 minute more. Transfer to a plate. Fill the lower half of the "tortilla" with the broccoli mixture and top with the bacon. Carefully roll into a "burrito."

Shrimp Scampi Zoodles

Ingredients

• 4 to 6 medium zucchini (2 1/4 to 2 1/2 pounds), trimmed

• ½ teaspoon salt, divided

• 2 tablespoons butter

• 2 tablespoons extra-virgin olive oil, divided

• 1 tablespoon minced garlic

• ⅓ cup dry white wine

• 1 pound peeled and deveined raw shrimp (16 to 20 per pound), tails left on, if desired

• 1 tablespoon lemon juice

• ¼ cup chopped fresh parsley

• ¼ teaspoon ground pepper

• ¼ cup grated Parmesan cheese

• Lemon wedges for serving

Directions

• Using a spiral vegetable slicer or a vegetable peeler, cut zucchini lengthwise into long, thin strands or strips. Place the zucchini noodles in a colander and toss with 1/4 teaspoon salt. Let drain for 15 to 30 minutes, then gently squeeze to remove any excess liquid.

• Meanwhile, heat butter and 1 tablespoon oil in a large skillet over medium-high heat. Add garlic and cook, stirring, for 30 seconds. Carefully add wine and bring to a simmer. Add shrimp and cook, stirring, until the shrimp are pink and just cooked through, 3 to 4 minutes. Remove from heat and add lemon juice, parsley, pepper and the remaining 1/4 teaspoon salt; stir to combine. Transfer to a large bowl and set aside.

• Heat the remaining 1 tablespoon oil in the skillet over medium-high heat. Add zucchini and gently toss until hot, about 3 minutes. Pour the shrimp mixture over the zucchini and gently toss to combine. Serve sprinkled with Parmesan and a squeeze of lemon.

Vegan Burrito Bowls with Cauliflower Rice

Ingredients

• 1 recipe Beefless Ground Beef

• 1 (12 ounce) package frozen riced cauliflower

- 4 teaspoons olive oil

- 1 teaspoon no-salt-added taco seasoning

- 1 cup thinly sliced red cabbage

- 1 cup diced avocado

- ½ cup pico de gallo or salsa

- ¼ cup chopped fresh cilantro

Directions

- Prepare Beefless Ground Beef as directed.

- While the Beefless Ground Beef cooks, prepare riced cauliflower according to package directions. Toss with oil and taco seasoning.

- Divide the cauliflower among 4 single-serving containers with lids. Top each with 1/2 cup Beefless Ground Beef, 1/4 cup each cabbage and avocado, 2 tablespoons pico de gallo (or salsa) and 1 tablespoon cilantro. Seal the containers and refrigerate until ready to eat.

Pork Chops with Garlicky Broccoli

Ingredients

• 1 ½ pounds broccoli with stems, trimmed and cut into spears

• 6 tablespoons extra-virgin olive oil, divided

• 1 cup panko breadcrumbs, preferably whole-wheat

• ¼ cup grated Parmesan cheese, plus more for serving

• ¼ cup whole-wheat flour

• 1 large egg, lightly beaten

• 4 (4 ounce) boneless pork chops, trimmed

• ¾ teaspoon salt, divided

• 1 teaspoon lemon juice

• 4 cloves garlic, thinly sliced

• ¼ teaspoon crushed red pepper

• 2 tablespoons red-wine vinegar

• 1 sprig Chopped fresh thyme for garnish

Directions

• Position rack in upper third of oven; preheat broiler to high. Line a rimmed baking sheet with foil.

• Toss broccoli with 1 1/2 tablespoons oil on the prepared pan and spread in an even layer. Broil, stirring once, until charred in spots, about 10 minutes. Transfer to a bowl and set aside.

• Meanwhile, combine breadcrumbs and Parmesan in a shallow dish. Place flour in another shallow dish and egg in a third shallow dish. Sprinkle pork with 1/4 teaspoon salt, then dredge in the flour, shaking off excess; dip in the egg, letting excess drip off; and coat with the breadcrumb mixture.

• Heat 3 tablespoons oil in a large nonstick skillet over medium-high heat. Add the pork and cook, turning once, until golden brown and an instant-read thermometer inserted in the thickest portion registers 145 degrees F, about 6 minutes total. (If the pork is browning too quickly, reduce heat to medium.) Transfer to a plate and drizzle with lemon juice. Tent with foil.

• Wipe the pan clean. Add the remaining 1 1/2 tablespoons oil, garlic and crushed red pepper and cook over low heat, stirring, until the garlic is sizzling, about 3 minutes. Remove from heat and stir in vinegar and the remaining 1/2 teaspoon salt. Drizzle over the reserved broccoli and toss to coat. Serve the pork and broccoli with more Parmesan and thyme, if desired.

Chicken Florentine

Ingredients

• 2 tablespoons extra-virgin olive oil, divided

• 1 pound chicken breast, thinly sliced

• ½ teaspoon salt, divided

• ½ teaspoon ground pepper, divided

• ¼ cup finely chopped shallot

• 2 large cloves garlic, minced

• ⅓ cup dry white wine

• 1 pound baby spinach

• ⅓ cup heavy cream

• 2 teaspoons cornstarch

Directions

• Heat 1 tablespoon oil in a large skillet over medium-high heat. Season chicken with 1/4 teaspoon each salt and pepper. Add to the pan and cook, turning once, until just cooked through, 5 to 7 minutes. Transfer to a plate and tent with foil to keep warm.

• Reduce heat to medium. Add the remaining 1 tablespoon oil, shallot and garlic to the pan. Cook, stirring, until fragrant, about 30 seconds. Add wine, scraping up any browned bits. Add spinach in batches and cook, stirring often, until wilted, 3 to 5 minutes. Whisk cream, cornstarch and the remaining 1/4 teaspoon each salt and pepper in a measuring cup. Stir into the spinach and cook until thickened, about 2 minutes more. Serve with the chicken.

Vegan Burrito Bowls with Cauliflower Rice

Ingredients

• 1 recipe Beefless Ground Beef

• 1 (12 ounce) package frozen riced cauliflower

• 4 teaspoons olive oil

• 1 teaspoon no-salt-added taco seasoning

• 1 cup thinly sliced red cabbage

• 1 cup diced avocado

• ½ cup pico de gallo or salsa

• ¼ cup chopped fresh cilantro

Directions

• Prepare Beefless Ground Beef as directed.

• While the Beefless Ground Beef cooks, prepare riced cauliflower according to package directions. Toss with oil and taco seasoning.

• Divide the cauliflower among 4 single-serving containers with lids. Top each with 1/2 cup Beefless Ground Beef, 1/4 cup each cabbage and avocado, 2 tablespoons pico de gallo (or salsa) and 1 tablespoon cilantro. Seal the containers and refrigerate until ready to eat.

Superfood Chopped Salad with Salmon & Creamy Garlic Dressing

Ingredients

• 1 pound salmon fillet

• ½ cup low-fat plain yogurt

• ¼ cup mayonnaise

• 2 tablespoons lemon juice

• 2 tablespoons grated Parmesan cheese

• 1 tablespoon finely chopped fresh parsley

• 1 tablespoon snipped fresh chives

• 2 teaspoons reduced-sodium tamari or soy sauce

• 1 medium clove garlic, minced

- ¼ teaspoon ground pepper

- 8 cups chopped curly kale

- 2 cups chopped broccoli

- 2 cups chopped red cabbage

- 2 cups finely diced carrots

- ½ cup sunflower seeds, toasted

Directions

- Arrange rack in upper third of oven. Preheat broiler to high. Line a baking sheet with foil.

- Place salmon on the prepared baking sheet, skin-side down. Broil, rotating the pan from front to back once, until the salmon is opaque in the center, 8 to 12 minutes. Cut into 4 portions.

- Meanwhile, whisk yogurt, mayonnaise, lemon juice, Parmesan, parsley, chives, tamari (or soy sauce), garlic and pepper in a small bowl.

• Combine kale, broccoli, cabbage, carrots and sunflower seeds in a large bowl. Add 3/4 cup of the dressing and toss to coat. Divide the salad among 4 dinner plates and top each with a piece of salmon and about 1 tablespoon of the remaining dressing.

Soy-Lime Beef & Cabbage Salad

Ingredients

• 4 cups packaged shredded broccoli slaw mix

• 3 cups packaged shredded cabbage with carrot (coleslaw mix)

• 3 medium red sweet peppers, cut into bite-size strips

• ¾ cup bias-sliced snow pea pods

• ½ cup thinly sliced red onion

• ½ cup light mayonnaise

• ⅓ cup light Asian salad dressing

• 3 tablespoons rice vinegar

- 2 tablespoons lime juice

- 2 tablespoons reduced-sodium soy sauce

- Nonstick cooking spray

- 1 pound lean ground beef (95% lean)

- ½ cup sliced green onions

- ¼ cup fresh cilantro leaves

- 1 jalapeño chile pepper, seeded (if desired) and sliced (Optional)

Directions

- In a large bowl combine the broccoli slaw mix, cabbage, sweet peppers, snow pea pods and red onion. Add mayonnaise and Asian dressing; stir to coat.

- In a small bowl combine the rice vinegar, lime juice and soy sauce.

- Coat a large nonstick skillet with cooking spray; heat skillet over medium heat. Add ground beef; cook until browned.

Drain off fat. Stir in soy mixture; cook until liquid is nearly evaporated. Remove from heat. Stir in green onions.

• Serve meat mixture over slaw mixture. Top with cilantro and, if desired, jalapeño pepper.

Guacamole Chicken

Ingredients

• 1 medium avocado

• 2 teaspoons chopped pimientos

• 1 teaspoon lime juice

• Pinch of salt plus 1/2 teaspoon, divided

• Pinch of ground pepper plus 1/2 teaspoon, divided

• 2 8-ounce boneless, skinless chicken breasts, halved

• ½ teaspoon garlic powder

• 1 tablespoon extra-virgin olive oil

• ½ cup shredded Monterey Jack cheese (1 ounce)

• 2 tablespoons chopped fresh cilantro

Directions

• Place avocado in a medium bowl; mash with a fork until smooth with some chunks remaining. Stir in pimientos, lime juice, a pinch of salt and a pinch of pepper. Set aside.

• Sprinkle chicken with the remaining 1/2 teaspoon salt, the remaining 1/2 teaspoon pepper and garlic powder. Heat oil in a large skillet over medium-high heat. Add the chicken and reduce heat to medium. Cook, turning once, until just cooked through, 4 to 6 minutes per side. Top with cheese; cover and continue cooking until the cheese has melted, about 2 minutes more. Transfer the chicken to a serving platter and top with the guacamole. Garnish with cilantro.

Mexican Cauliflower Rice

Ingredients

• 4 cups small cauliflower florets

• 3 tablespoons avocado oil

- ½ cup chopped onion

- 1 medium jalapeño pepper, finely chopped

- ¼ cup no-salt-added crushed tomatoes or tomato sauce

- ½ teaspoon ground cumin

- ½ teaspoon salt

- Chopped fresh cilantro for garnish

- Lime wedges for garnish

Directions

- Pulse cauliflower in a food processor until broken down into rice-size pieces.

- Heat oil in a large skillet over medium-high heat. Add onion and jalapeño; cook, stirring, until softened and beginning to brown, 2 to 5 minutes. Add the cauliflower, tomatoes, cumin and salt; continue cooking, stirring, until the cauliflower is soft, 4 to 5 minutes more. Garnish with cilantro, if desired, and serve with lime wedges.

Roasted Broccoli with Lemon-Garlic Vinaigrette

Ingredients

• 2 small broccoli crowns (about 8 ounces each)

• 4 tablespoons extra-virgin olive oil, divided

• ¼ teaspoon salt plus 1/8 teaspoon, divided

• 1 teaspoon lemon zest

• 1 tablespoon lemon juice

• 1 clove garlic, finely grated

• ⅛ teaspoon ground pepper

Directions

• Preheat oven to 425 degrees F.

• Slice broccoli crowns in half. Toss with 2 tablespoons oil and 1/4 teaspoon salt in a large bowl. Place cut-side down on a baking sheet. Roast until the stems are tender and browned, 25 to 30 minutes.

• Meanwhile, combine lemon zest, lemon juice, garlic, pepper and the remaining 1/8 teaspoon salt in a small bowl. Slowly whisk in the remaining 2 tablespoons oil. Drizzle the vinaigrette over the roasted broccoli.

Cauliflower Mac & Cheese

Ingredients

• 8 cups bite-size cauliflower florets (from 1-2 heads)

• 1 ¾ cups reduced-fat milk, divided

• 2 tablespoons cornstarch

• 2 cups shredded extra-sharp Cheddar cheese

• 8 ounces reduced-fat cream cheese, cut into pieces

• ½ teaspoon salt

• ⅛ teaspoon ground pepper

• Chopped fresh chives or parsley for garnish

Directions

61

• Cook cauliflower in a large pot of boiling water until just tender, 4 to 6 minutes. Drain.

• Meanwhile, heat 1 1/2 cups milk in a large heavy saucepan over medium-high heat until steaming. Whisk the remaining 1/4 cup milk and cornstarch in a small bowl until smooth; add to the hot milk and cook, whisking constantly, until the sauce simmers and thickens, 2 to 3 minutes. Remove from heat and stir in Cheddar and cream cheese until melted. Stir in salt and pepper. Add the cauliflower and stir to combine. Garnish with chives (or parsley), if desired.

Broiled Ginger-Lime Chicken

Ingredients

• 6 large or 12 small bone-in chicken thighs (2 1/2-3 pounds), skin removed

• ¼ cup finely chopped scallions

• 2 tablespoons finely chopped fresh ginger

• 2 tablespoons canola oil

• 1 tablespoon lime zest

• 2 tablespoons lime juice

• 1 teaspoon ground cinnamon

• 1 teaspoon salt

• ½ teaspoon ground pepper

• ½ teaspoon freshly grated nutmeg

• ⅛ teaspoon cayenne pepper

Directions

• Line a broiler pan or rimmed baking sheet with foil and coat with cooking spray.

• Pat chicken dry. Place on the prepared pan, skinned side up. Mix scallions, ginger, oil, lime zest and juice, cinnamon, salt, pepper, nutmeg and cayenne and spread on the chicken. Cover and refrigerate for 2 to 24 hours.

• Preheat broiler to high.

• Broil the chicken on the pan until an instant-read thermometer inserted in the thickest part registers 165 degrees F, 15 to 25 minutes.

Tequila Guacamole

Ingredients

• ¼ cup finely chopped white onion

• 3 tablespoons finely chopped jalapeño, seeds removed

• ¼ cup chopped tomato, seeds removed

• 1 tablespoon fresh lime juice

• 1 tablespoon silver tequila

• ⅜ teaspoon kosher salt

• 2 medium avocados

• Tortilla chips for serving

Directions

• Combine onion, jalapeño, tomato, lime juice, tequila and salt in a medium bowl.

• Add avocados and mash with a fork or potato masher to the desired consistency. Serve with tortilla chips.

Slow-Cooker Vegetable Soup

Ingredients

- 1 medium onion, chopped

- 2 medium carrots, chopped

- 2 stalks celery, chopped

- 12 ounces fresh green beans, cut into 1/2-inch pieces

- 4 cups chopped kale

- 2 medium zucchini, chopped

- 4 Roma tomatoes, seeded and chopped

- 2 cloves garlic, minced

- 2 (15 ounce) cans no-salt-added cannellini or other white beans, rinsed

- 4 cups low-sodium chicken broth or low-sodium vegetable broth

- 1 Parmesan rind (optional)

- 2 teaspoons salt

- ½ teaspoon ground pepper

- 2 teaspoons red-wine vinegar

- 8 teaspoons prepared pesto

Directions

- Combine onion, carrots, celery, green beans, kale, zucchini, tomatoes, garlic, white beans, broth, Parmesan rind (if using), salt and pepper in a 6-quart or larger slow cooker. Cover and cook on High for 4 hours or Low for 6 hours.

- Remove Parmesan rind, if using. Stir in vinegar and top each serving of soup with 1 teaspoon pesto.

Spicy Slaw Bowls with Shrimp & Edamame

Ingredients

- Spicy Cabbage Slaw

- 2 cups frozen shelled edamame, thawed

- 1 medium avocado, diced

- ½ medium lime, juiced

- 12 ounces peeled cooked shrimp

Directions

- Prepare Spicy Cabbage Slaw. Add edamame; toss and set aside.

- Toss avocado with lime juice in a small bowl.

- Divide the slaw mixture among 4 containers. Top each with 1/4 of the shrimp (about 3 ounces) and 1/4 of the avocado. Cover and refrigerate until ready to eat.

Taco-Stuffed Zucchini

Ingredients

- 2 large zucchini

- 1 tablespoon avocado oil

- ¾ pound lean ground beef

- 1 medium tomato, chopped

- 1 bunch scallions, sliced

- 1 tablespoon chili powder

- 2 teaspoons ground cumin

- ¾ teaspoon salt, divided

- ½ teaspoon garlic powder

- ¼ teaspoon ground pepper

- 8 tablespoons shredded Monterey Jack cheese

- 1 cup shredded romaine lettuce

- 1 avocado, chopped

- 4 tablespoons Pico de gallo

Directions

- Cut each zucchini in half lengthwise. Cut a thin slice off the bottoms so that each half sits flat. Scoop out the pulp, leaving a 1/4-inch shell. Chop the pulp.

• Heat oil in a large skillet over medium-high heat. Add beef, tomato, scallions, chili powder, cumin, 1/2 teaspoon salt and garlic powder. Cook, breaking the beef into small pieces, until no longer pink, 5 to 6 minutes. Stir in the chopped pulp.

• Meanwhile, place the prepared zucchini halves in a microwave-safe dish; sprinkle with the remaining 1/4 teaspoon salt and pepper. Cover and microwave on High until tender-crisp, 2 to 3 minutes. Uncover.

• Position rack in the upper third of the oven. Preheat broiler to high. Place the zucchini halves on a baking sheet. Divide the beef filling among the zucchini halves and sprinkle each half with 2 tablespoons cheese. Broil until the cheese is melted, about 2 minutes. Serve with lettuce, avocado and pico de gallo, if desired.

Cheesy Spinach-&-Artichoke Stuffed Spaghetti Squash

Ingredients

- 1 (2 1/2 to 3 pound) spaghetti squash, cut in half lengthwise and seeds removed

- 3 tablespoons water, divided

- 1 (5 ounce) package baby spinach

- 1 (10 ounce) package frozen artichoke hearts, thawed and chopped

- 4 ounces reduced-fat cream cheese, cubed and softened

- ½ cup grated Parmesan cheese, divided

- ¼ teaspoon salt

- ¼ teaspoon ground pepper

- Crushed red pepper & chopped fresh basil for garnish

Directions

- Place squash cut-side down in a microwave-safe dish; add 2 tablespoons water. Microwave, uncovered, on High until tender, 10 to 15 minutes. (Alternatively, place squash halves cut-side down on a rimmed baking sheet. Bake at 400 degrees F until tender, 40 to 50 minutes.)

• Meanwhile, combine spinach and the remaining 1 tablespoon water in a large skillet over medium heat. Cook, stirring occasionally, until wilted, 3 to 5 minutes. Drain and transfer to a large bowl.

• Position rack in upper third of oven; preheat broiler.

• Use a fork to scrape the squash from the shells into the bowl. Place the shells on a baking sheet. Stir artichoke hearts, cream cheese, 1/4 cup Parmesan, salt and pepper into the squash mixture. Divide it between the squash shells and top with the remaining 1/4 cup Parmesan. Broil until the cheese is golden brown, about 3 minutes. Sprinkle with crushed red pepper and basil, if desired.

Zucchini Enchiladas

Ingredients

• 2 tablespoons extra-virgin olive oil

• 1 medium onion, chopped

• 1 poblano pepper, seeded and chopped

- ¼ teaspoon salt

- 12 ounces cooked chicken breast, shredded (about 3 cups)

- 1 cup shredded Mexican-blend cheese, divided

- 1 (15 ounce) can enchilada sauce (1 1/2 cups), divided

- 3 medium zucchini (about 1 pound), trimmed

- ⅓ cup sour cream

- 3 tablespoons reduced-fat milk

- 1 cup shredded romaine lettuce

- ½ cup chopped fresh cilantro

Directions

- Preheat oven to 425 degrees F. Heat oil in a large skillet over medium-high heat. Add onion, poblano and salt. Cook, stirring frequently, until the vegetables have softened and are beginning to brown, about 6 minutes. Reduce heat to medium if vegetables start to burn. Transfer to a large bowl. Add chicken, 1/2 cup cheese and 1/2 cup enchilada sauce. Stir to combine; set aside.

• Using a vegetable peeler or mandolin slicer, slice zucchini lengthwise into thin strips (see Tip). Discard any uneven and broken pieces. You should end up with 48 slices.

• Spread 1/4 cup enchilada sauce on the bottom of a 9-by-13-inch baking dish. Lay three strips of zucchini on a clean work surface, overlapping the edges by 1/4 inch or so. Place 2 generous tablespoons of the chicken filling across the middle of the zucchini strips. Gently roll the zucchini strips around the filling and place seam-side down in the prepared dish. Repeat with the remaining zucchini strips and filling. (You should have 16 enchiladas.) Top the zucchini rolls with the remaining 3/4 cup enchilada sauce and 1/2 cup cheese.

• Bake until the sauce is bubbling and the cheese is melted, 20 to 25 minutes.

• Meanwhile, whisk sour cream and milk together in a small bowl. When the enchiladas have finished baking, top with lettuce and cilantro. Drizzle the sour cream mixture over the top.

Classic Beef Stroganoff

Ingredients

- 1 ¼ pounds beef stew meat

- 2 teaspoons vegetable oil

- 2 ½ cups sliced fresh mushrooms

- ½ cup sliced green onions (4) or chopped onion (1 medium)

- 1 bay leaf

- 2 cloves garlic, minced

- ½ teaspoon dried oregano, crushed

- ¼ teaspoon salt

- ¼ teaspoon dried thyme, crushed

- ¼ teaspoon black pepper

- 1 ½ cups 50% less sodium beef broth

- ¼ cup dry sherry

- 1 (8 ounce) carton light sour cream

- ⅓ cup all-purpose flour

• ¼ cup water

• Sauteed zucchini "noodles" or hot cooked whole-wheat pasta

• 1 sprig Snipped fresh parsley or basil

Directions

• Cut up any large pieces of meat. In a large nonstick skillet cook half of the meat in hot oil over medium-high heat until brown. Using a slotted spoon, remove meat from skillet. Repeat with the remaining meat. Drain off fat. Set meat aside.

• In a 3 1/2- or 4-quart slow cooker combine mushrooms, green onions, bay leaf, garlic, oregano, salt, thyme, and pepper. Add meat. Pour broth and sherry over mixture in cooker.

• Cover and cook on low-heat setting for 8 to 10 hours or on high-heat setting for 4 to 5 hours. Remove and discard bay leaf.

• If using low-heat setting, turn to high-heat setting. In a medium bowl stir together sour cream, flour, and the water until smooth. Gradually stir about 1 cup of the hot broth into sour cream mixture. Return sour cream mixture to cooker; stir to combine. Cover and cook about 30 minutes more or until thickened and bubbly. Serve over sauteed zucchini and, if desired, sprinkle with parsley.

Pork Chops with Balsamic Sweet Onions

Ingredients

• 4 boneless pork loin chops or cutlets, about 1/2 inch thick, trimmed (1-1 1/4 pounds total)

• ¾ teaspoon kosher salt

• ½ teaspoon ground pepper

• 1 tablespoon extra-virgin olive oil

• 2 cups thinly sliced sweet onions

• 1 teaspoon chopped fresh thyme

- ½ cup unsalted chicken broth

- ½ cup water

- ¼ cup golden raisins

- 3 tablespoons balsamic vinegar

- 1 tablespoon butter

- 1 tablespoon chopped flat-leaf parsley

Directions

• Sprinkle pork with salt and pepper. Heat oil in a large skillet over medium-high heat. Add the pork and cook, turning once, until browned, about 2 minutes per side. Reduce heat to medium and continue cooking until an instant-read thermometer registers 140 degrees F, 3 to 5 minutes more. Transfer the pork to a plate and tent with foil.

• Add onions and thyme to the pan; cook, stirring often, for 1 minute. Add broth and water; cover and cook for 5 minutes. Uncover and cook, stirring often, until the onions are soft and most of the liquid has evaporated, about 5 minutes. Stir in raisins and vinegar, scraping up any browned bits. Bring to a boil. Cook until thickened, about 3 minutes. Remove from heat and stir in butter. Serve the pork with the sauce, topped with parsley.

Miso Sweet Potatoes

Ingredients

• 1 ½ tablespoons butter, melted

• 2 teaspoons white miso

• ½ teaspoon ground pepper

• ¼ teaspoon salt

• 3 medium sweet potatoes (1 1/2 pounds total), sliced into 1-inch-thick rounds

• 1 tablespoon pure maple syrup

• 1 tablespoon cider vinegar

• 1 teaspoon chopped fresh rosemary

Directions

• Preheat oven to 425 degrees F. Line a large baking sheet with parchment paper.

• Combine butter, miso, pepper and salt in a large bowl. Add sweet potato slices and toss to coat. Arrange them in a single layer on the baking sheet; scrape any remaining butter-miso mixture over them. Roast the sweet potatoes, flipping once, until lightly browned and tender, about 30 minutes.

• Whisk maple syrup and vinegar in a small bowl. Drizzle over the sweet potatoes. Serve sprinkled with rosemary.

Chicken Satay Bowls with Spicy Peanut Sauce

Ingredients

• 1 recipe Thai Chicken Satay with Spicy Peanut Sauce

• 6 cups thinly sliced Savoy or green cabbage

• ½ cup thinly sliced red bell pepper

• ½ cup matchstick-cut carrots

- ¼ cup finely chopped green onion

- 2 tablespoons toasted sesame seeds

Directions

- Prepare Thai Chicken Satay with Spicy Peanut Sauce as directed. Remove the chicken from the skewers and cut into strips. Divide the sauce among 4 small condiment containers with lids and refrigerate until ready to use.

- To prepare slaw: Toss cabbage, bell pepper, carrots and green onion in a large bowl.

- Divide the slaw among 4 single-serving containers with lids. Top each with one-fourth of the chicken and 1/2 tablespoon sesame seeds. Dress with the reserved sauce just before serving.

Philly Cheesesteak Stuffed Peppers

Ingredients

- 2 large bell peppers, halved lengthwise, seeds removed

- 1 tablespoon extra-virgin olive oil

- 1 large onion, halved and sliced

- 1 (8 ounce) package mushrooms, thinly sliced

- 12 ounces top round steak, thinly sliced

- 1 tablespoon Italian seasoning

- ½ teaspoon ground pepper

- ¼ teaspoon salt

- 1 tablespoon Worcestershire sauce

- 4 slices provolone cheese

Directions

- Preheat oven to 375 degrees F.

- Place pepper halves on a rimmed baking sheet. Bake until tender but still holding their shape, about 30 minutes.

- Meanwhile, heat oil in a large skillet over medium heat. Add onion and cook, stirring, until starting to brown, 4 to 5 minutes. Add mushrooms and cook, stirring, until they're softened and release their juices, about 5 minutes more. Add steak, Italian seasoning, pepper and salt; cook, stirring, until the steak is just cooked through, 3 to 5 minutes more. Remove from heat and stir in Worcestershire.

• Preheat broiler to high. Divide the filling between the pepper halves and top each with a slice of cheese. Broil 5 inches from the heat until the cheese is melted and lightly browned, 2 to 3 minutes.

Two-Ingredient Banana Pancakes

Ingredients

• 2 large eggs

• 1 medium banana

Directions

• Puree eggs and banana in a blender until smooth.

• Lightly oil a large nonstick skillet (see Tip) and heat over medium heat. Using 2 tablespoons of batter for each pancake, drop 4 mounds of batter into the pan. Cook until bubbles appear on the surface and the edges look dry, 2 to 4 minutes. Using a thin spatula, gently flip the pancakes and cook until browned on the bottom, 1 to 2 minutes more. Transfer the pancakes to a plate. Lightly oil the pan again and repeat with the remaining batter.

Hummus-Crusted Chicken

Ingredients

• ⅔ cup prepared hummus

• 1 teaspoon ground cumin

• 1 teaspoon lemon zest (from 1 lemon)

• ½ teaspoon paprika

• ¼ teaspoon salt

- ½ teaspoon ground pepper

- 4 (6 ounce) boneless, skinless chicken breasts

- ¼ cup toasted sesame seeds

- 2 tablespoons chopped fresh parsley

- Lemon wedges for serving

Directions

- Preheat oven to 400 degrees F. Line a rimmed baking sheet with foil.

- Whisk hummus, cumin, lemon zest, paprika, salt and pepper in a small bowl. Spread the mixture evenly on both sides of chicken breasts. Sprinkle both sides with sesame seeds, pressing gently to adhere. Place on the prepared pan.

- Roast the chicken until an instant-read thermometer inserted in the thickest part registers 160 degrees F, about 20 minutes. Let stand for 5 minutes (the temperature will increase to 165 degrees F). Sprinkle with parsley and serve with lemon wedges.

Balsamic & Parmesan Broccoli

Ingredients

- 2 tablespoons extra-virgin olive oil, divided

- 6 cups broccoli florets (about 12 ounces)

- 1 small shallot, sliced

- 1 tablespoon minced garlic

- 1 tablespoon white balsamic vinegar

- ¼ teaspoon salt

- ¼ teaspoon ground black pepper

- ⅓ cup finely shredded Parmesan cheese

Directions

- Heat 1 tablespoon oil in a large flat-bottom carbon-steel wok over medium-high heat. Add broccoli and cook, stirring, until browned in spots, about 4 minutes. Reduce heat to medium. Push the broccoli to the sides and add the remaining 1 tablespoon oil, shallot, garlic, vinegar, salt and pepper; cook, stirring often, until the broccoli is tender, about 3 minutes more. Remove from heat and sprinkle with Parmesan. Cover and let stand until the cheese is melted, 1 to 2 minutes.

Egg Salad Lettuce Wraps

Ingredients

- ¼ cup plain nonfat Greek yogurt

- 1 tablespoon mayonnaise

- ½ teaspoon Dijon mustard

- Pinch of salt

- Ground pepper to taste

- 3 hard-boiled eggs, peeled

- 2 stalks celery, minced

- 2 tablespoons minced red onion

- 2 or 3 large iceberg lettuce leaves

- 1 tablespoon chopped fresh basil

- 2 carrots, peeled and cut into sticks

Directions

- Whisk yogurt, mayonnaise, mustard, salt and pepper in a medium bowl. Discard one egg yolk. Chop the remaining eggs and transfer to the bowl. Add celery and onion and stir to combine. Cut lettuce leaves in half and double-layer them to make 2 lettuce wraps. Divide the egg salad among the wraps and top with basil. Serve with carrot sticks on the side.

Spaghetti Squash with Roasted Tomatoes, Beans & Almond Pesto

Ingredients

Almond Pesto

- 2 cups fresh basil leaves

87

- 1 cup fresh parsley leaves

- ½ cup grated Parmesan cheese

- ⅓ cup whole raw almonds

- 1 clove garlic

- 1 ½ tablespoons red-wine vinegar

- ¼ teaspoon kosher salt

- ¼ teaspoon ground pepper

- ¼ cup extra-virgin olive oil

- ¼ cup water

Spaghetti Squash & Vegetables

- 1 3-pound spaghetti squash

- ¼ cup water

- 2 pints grape tomatoes, halved

- 1 tablespoon extra-virgin olive oil

- ¼ teaspoon kosher salt

- ¼ teaspoon ground pepper

• 1 cup canned cannellini beans, rinsed

Directions

• To prepare pesto: Pulse basil, parsley, Parmesan, almonds, garlic, vinegar and 1/4 teaspoon each salt and pepper in a food processor until coarsely chopped, scraping down the sides. With the motor running, add 1/4 cup oil; process until well combined.

• Add water to the pesto in the food processor; pulse to combine.

• To prepare squash & vegetables: Preheat oven to 400 degrees F. Line a rimmed baking sheet with foil.

• Halve squash lengthwise and scoop out the seeds. Place cut-side down in a microwave-safe dish and add water. Microwave on High until the flesh can be easily scraped with a fork, about 15 minutes.

• Meanwhile, toss tomatoes with oil, salt and pepper in a large bowl. Transfer to the prepared baking sheet. Roast until soft and wrinkled, 10 to 12 minutes. Remove from the oven. Add beans and stir to combine.

• Scrape the squash flesh into the bowl and divide among 4 plates. Top each portion with some of the tomato-bean mixture and about 3 tablespoons pesto sauce.

Easy Loaded Baked Omelet Muffins

Ingredients

• 3 slices bacon, chopped

• 2 cups finely chopped broccoli

• 4 scallions, sliced

• 8 large eggs

• 1 cup shredded Cheddar cheese

• ½ cup low-fat milk

• ½ teaspoon salt

• ½ teaspoon ground pepper

Directions

• Preheat oven to 325 degrees F. Coat a 12-cup muffin tin with cooking spray.

• Cook bacon in a large skillet over medium heat until crisp, 4 to 5 minutes. Remove with a slotted spoon to a paper towel-lined plate, leaving the bacon fat in the pan. Add broccoli and scallions and cook, stirring, until soft, about 5 minutes. Remove from heat and let cool for 5 minutes.

• Meanwhile, whisk eggs, cheese, milk, salt and pepper in a large bowl. Stir in the bacon and broccoli mixture. Divide the egg mixture among the prepared muffin cups.

• Bake until firm to the touch, 25 to 30 minutes. Let stand for 5 minutes before removing from the muffin tin.

Korean Steak, Kimchi & Cauliflower Rice Bowls

Ingredients

- 2 large eggs

- 4 tablespoons toasted sesame oil, divided

- 6 cups riced cauliflower

- 2 scallions, sliced, greens and whites separated

- 1 tablespoon minced ginger

- ¼ teaspoon salt

- 1 pound sirloin steak, thinly sliced

- ¼ cup gochujang

- 2 tablespoons toasted sesame seeds

- 1 cup shredded carrots

- ½ cup kimchi

- 1 ounce Sliced radishes for garnish

Directions

- Bring a medium saucepan of water to a boil over high heat. Set a bowl of ice water near the stove. Using a spoon, gently lower eggs into the boiling water. Reduce heat to maintain a rapid simmer. Cook for 7 minutes. Transfer the eggs to the ice bath and let cool for 5 minutes. Peel the eggs and slice in half.

• Meanwhile, heat 2 tablespoons oil in a large skillet over medium-high heat. Add cauliflower, scallion whites, ginger and salt. Cook, stirring frequently, until the cauliflower is softened, about 5 minutes. Transfer to a bowl and cover to keep warm. Wash and dry the pan.

• Heat the remaining 2 tablespoons oil in the pan over medium-high heat. Add steak and cook, stirring, until no longer pink, 2 to 4 minutes. Remove from heat and stir in gochujang and sesame seeds.

• To assemble, divide the cauliflower among 4 bowls. Top with the steak, carrots, kimchi, half an egg, scallion greens and radishes, if desired.

Zucchini Noodles with Quick Turkey Bolognese

Ingredients

- 3 cups Quick Turkey Meat Sauce

- 8 cups zucchini noodles (from 3 medium zucchini)

- ½ cup grated Parmesan cheese

Directions

- Prepare Quick Turkey Meat Sauce as directed.

- As the sauce cooks, divide zucchini noodles among 4 single-serving containers with lids (about 2 cups per container).

- Add 3/4 cup of the sauce and 2 tablespoons Parmesan to each container. Seal and refrigerate for up to 4 days.

- To reheat, vent the lid and microwave on High until the sauce is steaming and the noodles are tender, 2 1/2 to 3 minutes.

One-Pot Garlicky Shrimp & Spinach

Ingredients

- 3 tablespoons extra-virgin olive oil, divided

- 6 medium cloves garlic, sliced, divided

- 1 pound spinach

- ¼ teaspoon salt plus 1/8 teaspoon, divided

- 1 ½ teaspoons lemon zest

- 1 tablespoon lemon juice

- 1 pound shrimp (21-30 count), peeled and deveined

- ¼ teaspoon crushed red pepper

- 1 tablespoon finely chopped fresh parsley

Directions

• Heat 1 tablespoon oil in a large pot over medium heat. Add half the garlic and cook until beginning to brown, 1 to 2 minutes. Add spinach and 1/4 teaspoon salt and toss to coat. Cook, stirring once or twice, until mostly wilted, 3 to 5 minutes. Remove from heat and stir in lemon juice. Transfer to a bowl and keep warm.

- Increase heat to medium-high and add the remaining 2 tablespoons oil to the pot. Add the remaining garlic and cook until beginning to brown, 1 to 2 minutes. Add shrimp, crushed red pepper and the remaining 1/8 teaspoon salt; cook, stirring, until the shrimp are just cooked through, 3 to 5 minutes more. Serve the shrimp over the spinach, sprinkled with lemon zest and parsley.

CONCLUSION

Adopting a 1200 calorie low-carb diet can be an effective and sustainable approach to weight loss for many individuals. By limiting carbohydrates and focusing on nutrient-dense, high-protein foods, this meal plan helps create a calorie deficit without depriving the body of essential vitamins, minerals, and macronutrients.

The key to the success of this 1200 calorie low-carb diet lies in its balanced approach. Rather than eliminating carbohydrates entirely, as seen in more restrictive plans like keto, this meal plan aims to keep carb intake moderate while ensuring adequate fiber, vitamins, and minerals from sources like fruits, vegetables, and dairy. This helps prevent the unpleasant side effects that can sometimes arise from extremely low-carb diets, such as fatigue, constipation, and nutrient deficiencies.

One of the primary benefits of a 1200 calorie low-carb diet is its ability to promote satiety and curb hunger. By emphasizing protein-rich foods like lean meats, eggs, and Greek yogurt, this plan helps keep you feeling full and satisfied on fewer overall calories. The high-fiber content of low-carb vegetables and berries also contributes to this effect, slowing the digestive process and delaying the return of hunger pangs.

Additionally, the low-carb nature of this meal plan may help facilitate fat loss by encouraging the body to utilize stored fat as a fuel source, rather than relying primarily on glucose from carbohydrates. This metabolic shift, known as ketosis, can be an effective way to accelerate weight loss, especially when combined with regular physical activity.

However, it's important to note that the success of a 1200 calorie low-carb diet ultimately comes down to individual factors, such as one's starting weight, metabolism, and overall lifestyle. While many people may experience significant weight loss on this plan, others may find that a slightly higher calorie target or a more moderate carb restriction works better for their specific needs and preferences.

To ensure long-term sustainability, it's crucial to approach this 1200 calorie low-carb diet with a mindset of balance and moderation. Restrictive eating patterns that are overly rigid or lacking in variety can be difficult to maintain, leading to burnout and potential weight regain. Instead, focus on incorporating a wide range of nutrient-dense, low-carb foods that you genuinely enjoy, and find ways to make the diet fit seamlessly into your daily routine.

Additionally, regular physical activity, stress management, and adequate sleep are all important components of a successful weight loss journey. By addressing these lifestyle factors in conjunction with a 1200 calorie low-carb diet, you can create a holistic approach that supports both physical and mental well-being.

In conclusion, a 1200 calorie low-carb meal plan can be an effective and sustainable approach to weight loss for many individuals. By striking a balance between carbohydrate restriction and nutrient adequacy, this plan helps support fat loss while preserving overall health and well-being. However, it's essential to tailor the diet to your individual needs and preferences, and to incorporate it as part of a broader, holistic lifestyle approach to achieve long-lasting results.